Table of Contents

Chapter 1: Introduction to Fatty Liver

Welcome to the world of liver health and the journey towards understanding and managing fatty liver disease. In this chapter, we will delve into the intricate workings of the liver, explore the various aspects of fatty liver disease, and discover the crucial role that diet plays in its management and reversal. Prepare to embark on a captivating exploration of your liver's health and well-being.

1.1 Understanding Fatty Liver Disease:

The liver, our body's largest internal organ, is a powerhouse of vital functions. It acts as a filter, removing toxins from the bloodstream, producing bile to aid in digestion, and storing essential nutrients for energy. However, when fat begins to accumulate in the liver cells, it can lead to a condition known as fatty liver disease.

Fatty liver disease encompasses two main types: alcoholic fatty liver disease (AFLD) and non-alcoholic fatty liver disease (NAFLD). AFLD is caused by excessive alcohol consumption, while NAFLD is associated with factors such as obesity, insulin resistance, and metabolic syndrome. NAFLD has become increasingly prevalent in recent years, affecting millions of individuals worldwide.

1.2 Causes and Risk Factors:

While the exact causes of fatty liver disease are not fully understood, certain risk factors have been identified. Obesity, particularly excess abdominal fat, is strongly linked to NAFLD. Other risk factors include insulin resistance, type 2 diabetes, high blood pressure, high cholesterol levels, and a sedentary lifestyle. Genetic factors and certain medications can also contribute to the development of fatty liver disease.

1.3 Importance of Diet in Fatty Liver Management:

One of the most effective ways to manage and even reverse fatty liver disease is through dietary modifications. A well-balanced and nutrient-dense diet plays a crucial role in reducing liver fat, improving liver function, and promoting overall health. By making informed choices about what we eat, we can take control of our liver health and pave the way for a brighter future.

In the following chapters, we will explore the fundamentals of a fatty liver diet, learn about the key nutrients that support liver health, and discover the foods to avoid for optimal liver function. We will delve into the art of meal planning, providing you with practical tips and sample meal plans tailored to different dietary needs. Additionally, we will explore the essential foods that promote a healthy liver, including liver-friendly fruits and vegetables, lean protein sources, whole grains, and healthy fats.

Beyond diet, we will discuss the detrimental effects of substances such as alcohol, sugar, artificial sweeteners, and caffeine on the liver. It is crucial to understand the impact these substances can have on our liver health and make informed choices to minimize their consumption or avoid them altogether.

Lifestyle changes, including regular exercise, stress management, quality sleep, and smoking cessation, are also vital in supporting liver health. We will explore the scientific evidence behind these lifestyle factors and provide practical strategies for incorporating them into your daily routine.

Furthermore, we will delve into the world of supplements and explore the essential vitamins, minerals, and herbal remedies that can support liver health. It is important to note that while supplements can play a role, they should never replace a well-balanced diet or medical advice. We will provide guidance on using supplements safely and the importance of consulting with healthcare professionals.

To ensure that you stay on track with your liver health journey, we will discuss the importance of regular medical check-ups, liver function tests, and monitoring your progress. We will address common questions and misconceptions surrounding fatty liver disease and provide additional resources for further reading and support.

In conclusion, this chapter has provided an overview of fatty liver disease, its causes and risk factors, and the importance of diet in its management. The subsequent chapters will dive deeper into the practical aspects of a fatty liver diet, lifestyle changes, supplements, and monitoring your liver health. Get ready to transform your relationship with food, nurture your liver, and embark on a journey towards improved health and well-being.

Chapter 2: Fundamentals of a Fatty Liver Diet

Now that we have explored the basics of fatty liver disease, it's time to dive deeper into the fundamental principles of a fatty liver diet. In this chapter, we will unravel the secrets of a healthy liver diet, understand the key nutrients that support liver health, and uncover the foods to avoid for optimal liver function. Get ready to embark on a flavorful and nourishing journey towards healing your liver and improving your overall well-being.

2.1 Basics of a Healthy Liver Diet:

A healthy liver diet is centered around providing essential nutrients while minimizing the intake of harmful substances. It emphasizes whole, unprocessed foods that are rich in vitamins, minerals, antioxidants, and fiber. By adopting a liver-friendly eating plan, we can reduce inflammation, support liver function, and promote overall health.

To create a well-rounded liver diet, it is important to focus on the following principles:

a) Balance and Variety: Incorporate a variety of nutrient-dense foods from different food groups, including fruits, vegetables, whole grains, lean proteins, and healthy fats. Aim for a balance between carbohydrates, proteins, and fats to meet your body's nutritional needs.

b) Portion Control: Be mindful of portion sizes to maintain a healthy weight and prevent overeating. Listen to your body's hunger and fullness cues and practice mindful eating.

c) Hydration: Drink an adequate amount of water throughout the day to support liver function and flush out toxins. Limit the consumption of sugary beverages and opt for water, herbal teas, or infused water instead.

d) Cooking Methods: Choose healthier cooking methods such as baking, grilling, steaming, or sautéing instead of deep-frying or using excessive amounts of oil. This helps to reduce unnecessary fat and calorie intake.

2.2 Key Nutrients for Liver Health:

Now let's explore the key nutrients that play a vital role in supporting liver health:

a) Antioxidants: Antioxidants protect the liver from oxidative stress and inflammation. Include foods rich in antioxidants, such as berries, leafy greens, citrus fruits, cruciferous vegetables, and colorful fruits and vegetables.

b) Fiber: Fiber aids in digestion, helps maintain healthy blood sugar levels, and promotes a feeling of fullness. Include high-fiber foods like whole grains, legumes, fruits, vegetables, and nuts and seeds in your diet.

c) Omega-3 Fatty Acids: Omega-3 fatty acids have anti-inflammatory properties and may help reduce liver fat. Include fatty fish like salmon, sardines, and mackerel, as well as walnuts, chia seeds, and flaxseeds, as good sources of omega-3s.

d) Vitamin E: Vitamin E is an antioxidant that may protect liver cells from damage. Incorporate foods rich in vitamin E, such as nuts, seeds, spinach, and avocados.

e) B Vitamins: B vitamins, including folate, B6, and B12, are essential for liver health and metabolism. Include sources of B vitamins such as leafy greens, legumes, fortified cereals, eggs, and lean meats.

f) Selenium: Selenium is a mineral that supports liver health and acts as an antioxidant. Good sources of selenium include Brazil nuts, seafood, whole grains, and legumes.

g) Milk Thistle: Milk thistle is an herbal supplement that has been traditionally used to support liver health. Consult with a healthcare professional before incorporating milk thistle or any other herbal supplement into your diet.

2.3 Foods to Avoid for Fatty Liver:

While focusing on liver-friendly foods, it is equally important to be aware of the foods that can negatively impact liver health. Limit or avoid the following:

a) Alcohol: Excessive alcohol consumption is a leading cause of liver damage. If you have fatty liver disease, it is crucial to eliminate alcohol completely or significantly reduce your intake.

b) Added Sugars: Sugary foods and beverages contribute to weight gain, insulin resistance, and inflammation. Limit your consumption of sugary treats, sodas, fruit juices, and sweetened snacks.

c) Trans Fats: Trans fats are known to increase liver fat and inflammation. Avoid foods containing trans fats, such as fried foods, commercial baked goods, and processed snacks.

d) Saturated Fats: High intake of saturated fats can lead to inflammation and liver damage. Limit your consumption of fatty meats, full-fat dairy products, butter, and high-fat processed foods.

e) Sodium: Excess sodium can contribute to fluid retention and liver inflammation. Limit your intake of processed foods, canned soups, and salty snacks.

f) Refined Grains: Refined grains lack fiber and essential nutrients. Choose whole grains like brown rice, quinoa, whole wheat bread, and oats instead of refined grain products.

g) Added Sugary Drinks: Sugar-sweetened beverages, such as soda and energy drinks, can contribute to weight gain and liver damage. Opt for water, herbal tea, or naturally flavored water instead.

By understanding the basics of a healthy liver diet, the key nutrients that support liver health, and the foods to avoid, you are equipped with the knowledge to make informed choices and take control of your liver health. In the next chapter, we will explore the art of meal planning for fatty liver, providing you with practical tips and sample meal plans tailored to different dietary needs. Get ready to discover the joy of nourishing your body and nurturing your liver.

Chapter 3: Meal Planning for Fatty Liver

In this chapter, we will delve into the art of meal planning for fatty liver. By taking a thoughtful and strategic approach to your meals, you can optimize your nutrition, support liver health, and achieve your health goals. Get ready to explore the building blocks of a balanced meal, understand the importance of portion control and calorie management, and discover sample meal plans tailored to different dietary needs. It's time to create a roadmap to a healthier, happier liver.

3.1 Building a Balanced Meal:

A balanced meal consists of the right combination of nutrients to nourish your body and support liver health. Let's explore the building blocks of a balanced meal:

a) Protein: Include a source of lean protein in each meal, such as skinless chicken, turkey, fish, tofu, legumes, or low-fat dairy products. Protein is essential for tissue repair and helps stabilize blood sugar levels.

b) Vegetables: Fill half of your plate with a variety of non-starchy vegetables, such as leafy greens, broccoli, cauliflower, peppers, zucchini, and carrots. Vegetables are rich in fiber, vitamins, minerals, and antioxidants.

c) Whole Grains: Choose whole grains like brown rice, quinoa, whole wheat bread, and oats over refined grains. Whole grains provide fiber, vitamins, minerals, and sustained energy.

d) Healthy Fats: Incorporate sources of healthy fats into your meals, such as avocados, nuts, seeds, and olive oil. Healthy fats support liver function, promote satiety, and aid in the absorption of fat-soluble vitamins.

e) Fruits: Include a serving of fresh or frozen fruit with your meals for added vitamins, minerals, fiber, and natural sweetness.

f) Dairy or Dairy Alternatives: If you consume dairy, choose low-fat or fat-free options like skim milk, low-fat yogurt, or reduced-fat cheese. If you prefer dairy alternatives, opt for unsweetened plant-based milk or yogurt.

3.2 Portion Control and Calorie Management:

Portion control is key to maintaining a healthy weight and managing your calorie intake. Here are some tips to help you manage portion sizes:

a) Use smaller plates and bowls to create the illusion of a fuller plate.

b) Fill half of your plate with non-starchy vegetables, one-quarter with lean protein, and one-quarter with whole grains or starchy vegetables.

c) Be mindful of serving sizes and read nutrition labels to understand portion sizes.

d) Listen to your body's hunger and fullness cues. Eat until you are comfortably satisfied, not overly full.

e) Avoid distractions while eating, such as watching TV or using electronic devices. Focus on the taste and enjoyment of your food.

f) Practice portion control with higher-calorie foods like nuts, oils, and dressings, as they can contribute to excess calorie intake if consumed in large quantities.

Calorie management is crucial for weight management and liver health. While calorie needs vary depending on factors such as age, gender, activity level, and weight goals, it is important to consume an appropriate amount of calories to support your liver and overall health. Consulting with a registered dietitian or healthcare professional can help you determine your specific calorie needs.

3.3 Sample Meal Plans for Different Dietary Needs:

Now let's explore sample meal plans that can be adapted to different dietary needs and preferences:

a) Mediterranean-inspired Meal Plan:

   - Breakfast: Greek yogurt with berries and a sprinkle of nuts/seeds.

   - Snack: Carrot sticks with hummus.

   - Lunch: Grilled chicken breast salad with mixed greens, tomatoes, cucumbers, and olive oil vinaigrette.

   - Snack: Apple slices with almond butter.

   - Dinner: Baked salmon with quinoa and roasted vegetables.

   - Dessert: Greek yogurt with honey and a sprinkle of cinnamon.

b) Plant-based Meal Plan:

- Breakfast: Overnight chia pudding with almond milk, topped with mixed berries.

- Snack: Celery sticks with almond butter.

- Lunch: Chickpea and vegetable stir-fry with quinoa.

- Snack: Mixed nuts and seeds.

- Dinner: Roasted tofu with roasted sweet potatoes and steamed broccoli.

- Dessert: Baked apples with a sprinkle of cinnamon.

c) Low-carb Meal Plan:

- Breakfast: Vegetable omelet with spinach, mushrooms, and feta cheese.

- Snack: Hard-boiled eggs.

- Lunch: Grilled chicken salad with mixed greens, tomatoes, cucumbers, and olive oil dressing.

- Snack: Sliced cucumber with guacamole.

- Dinner: Baked salmon with steamed asparagus and cauliflower rice.

- Dessert: Berries with whipped coconut cream.

Remember, these sample meal plans are just starting points and can be customized to meet your specific dietary needs and preferences. Consider consulting with a registered dietitian to create a personalized meal plan that aligns with your goals and ensures optimal liver health.

In conclusion, this chapter has provided insight into the art of meal planning for fatty liver. By building balanced meals, practicing portion control, and managing calorie intake, you can optimize your nutrition, support your liver's health, and work towards achieving your health goals. Whether you follow a Mediterranean-inspired, plant-based, low-carb, or another dietary approach, there are endless possibilities for creating nourishing and delicious meals that promote a healthier liver and a vibrant life. In the next chapter, we will explore the essential foods for a healthy liver, including liver-friendly fruits and vegetables, lean protein sources, whole grains, and healthy fats. Get ready to embrace the power of nutritious foods and fuel your liver for optimal health.

Chapter 4: Essential Foods for a Healthy Liver

In this chapter, we will explore the essential foods for a healthy liver. Your diet plays a critical role in supporting liver health, and by incorporating liver-friendly foods into your meals, you can nourish your liver, reduce inflammation, and promote optimal functioning. Get ready to discover the power of fruits and vegetables, lean protein sources, whole grains, and healthy fats in promoting a vibrant and resilient liver.

4.1 Liver-Friendly Fruits and Vegetables:

Fruits and vegetables are packed with essential nutrients, antioxidants, and fiber, making them crucial components of a liver-friendly diet. Let's explore some liver-loving produce:

a) Berries: Berries like blueberries, strawberries, raspberries, and blackberries are rich in antioxidants that combat oxidative stress and reduce inflammation. Add them to your breakfast smoothies, yogurt bowls, or enjoy them as a refreshing snack.

b) Leafy Greens: Spinach, kale, Swiss chard, and other leafy greens are excellent sources of vitamins, minerals, and fiber. They also contain chlorophyll, which helps detoxify the liver. Incorporate leafy greens into salads, stir-fries, or sautés.

c) Cruciferous Vegetables: Broccoli, cauliflower, Brussels sprouts, and cabbage belong to the cruciferous vegetable family, known for their liver-protective properties. They contain compounds that support detoxification processes in the liver. Enjoy them steamed, roasted, or added to stir-fries.

d) Citrus Fruits: Oranges, grapefruits, lemons, and limes are rich in vitamin C and other antioxidants that aid in liver detoxification. Start your day with a glass of freshly squeezed citrus juice or add slices of citrus fruits to your water for a refreshing twist.

e) Apples: Apples contain pectin, a type of fiber that helps eliminate toxins from the digestive system. They also provide antioxidants and vitamins. Enjoy apples as a snack or incorporate them into salads or baked goods.

f) Beetroot: Beetroots are rich in antioxidants and contain betaine, which supports liver health. Enjoy roasted beetroots in salads or blend them into a vibrant beetroot smoothie.

g) Carrots: Carrots are rich in beta-carotene, a precursor to vitamin A, which supports liver function. Snack on carrot sticks, add them to salads, or include them in your favorite vegetable dishes.

These are just a few examples of liver-friendly fruits and vegetables. Aim to incorporate a variety of colorful produce into your meals to maximize the array of nutrients and antioxidants you consume.

4.2 Lean Protein Sources for Liver Health:

Protein is essential for the repair and regeneration of liver cells. Including lean protein sources in your diet ensures that your liver receives the building blocks it needs. Consider the following options:

a) Poultry: Skinless chicken breast and turkey breast are lean sources of protein. Grill, bake, or roast them and pair them with a side of vegetables or whole grains.

b) Fish: Fatty fish like salmon, sardines, and mackerel are not only excellent sources of protein but also provide omega-3 fatty acids, which have anti-inflammatory properties and may help reduce liver fat. Aim to incorporate fish into your diet at least twice a week.

c) Tofu and Tempeh: These plant-based protein sources are rich in amino acids and can be used in various dishes as meat alternatives. Experiment with different cooking methods and seasonings to enhance their flavors.

d) Legumes: Beans, lentils, and chickpeas are affordable, versatile, and rich in protein and fiber.

Include them in soups, stews, salads, or make delicious plant-based patties.

e) Low-Fat Dairy Products: If you consume dairy, choose low-fat or fat-free options like skim milk, low-fat yogurt, or reduced-fat cheese. Dairy products provide high-quality protein and essential nutrients. Opt for plain or Greek yogurt and avoid added sugars.

f) Eggs: Eggs are a nutrient-dense source of protein, vitamins, and minerals. Enjoy them boiled, scrambled, or in omelets, and combine them with vegetables for a nourishing meal.

Remember to prepare proteins using healthier cooking methods like grilling, baking, or steaming, rather than deep-frying or using excessive amounts of oil.

4.3 Whole Grains and Complex Carbohydrates:

Whole grains are a valuable source of fiber, vitamins, minerals, and complex carbohydrates. They provide sustained energy and support overall health, including liver health. Consider incorporating the following whole grains into your diet:

a) Brown Rice: Swap refined white rice for nutrient-rich brown rice. It provides more fiber, vitamins, and minerals, and has a lower glycemic index.

b) Quinoa: Quinoa is a complete protein source and a good alternative to refined grains. It is versatile and can be used in salads, stir-fries, or as a side dish.

c) Oats: Oats are packed with fiber and can help regulate blood sugar levels. Enjoy a warm bowl of oatmeal for breakfast or incorporate oats into baked goods.

d) Whole Wheat: Choose whole wheat bread, pasta, and wraps instead of their refined counterparts. Whole wheat products provide more fiber and nutrients.

e) Barley: Barley is a nutritious whole grain with a chewy texture. It can be used in soups, stews, salads, or as a side dish.

f) Buckwheat: Despite its name, buckwheat is not related to wheat and is gluten-free. It is rich in fiber and can be used to make delicious pancakes, noodles, or as a side dish.

Whole grains can be a part of your main meals or snacks. Experiment with different recipes to incorporate them into your diet.

4.4 Incorporating Healthy Fats into Your Diet:

Healthy fats are an essential component of a liver-friendly diet. They support the absorption of fat-soluble vitamins, provide energy, and help reduce inflammation. Include the following sources of healthy fats:

a) Avocados: Avocados are rich in monounsaturated fats, which can help lower LDL (bad) cholesterol levels. Enjoy avocado slices in salads, on toast, or as a creamy addition to smoothies.

b) Nuts and Seeds: Almonds, walnuts, flaxseeds, chia seeds, and hemp seeds are excellent sources of healthy fats, fiber, and antioxidants. Sprinkle them on salads, yogurt, or blend them into smoothies.

c) Olive Oil: Extra virgin olive oil is a staple of the Mediterranean diet and is rich in monounsaturated fats and antioxidants. Use it in salad dressings, for sautéing vegetables, or as a dip for whole grain bread.

d) Coconut Oil: While coconut oil is high in saturated fats, it contains medium-chain triglycerides (MCTs) that can be beneficial for the liver. Use it sparingly in cooking or baking.

e) Nut Butter: Opt for natural nut butter without added sugars or hydrogenated oils. Enjoy a spread of almond, peanut, or cashew butter on whole grain toast or use them as a dip for fruits or vegetables.

Remember that healthy fats should be consumed in moderation, as they are high in calories. Aim to include a variety of healthy fats in your meals and be mindful of portion sizes.

By incorporating liver-friendly fruits and vegetables, lean protein sources, whole grains, and healthy fats into your diet,

you can provide your liver with the essential nutrients it needs to thrive. Experiment with different recipes, flavors, and cooking methods to make your meals exciting and enjoyable.

Consider the following meal ideas that incorporate these liver-friendly foods:

a) Grilled salmon with a side of steamed broccoli and quinoa.

b) Chicken breast stir-fry with a colorful array of vegetables and brown rice.

c) Tofu and vegetable curry with whole wheat naan bread.

d) Spinach and berry salad topped with grilled chicken and a drizzle of olive oil dressing.

e) Lentil and vegetable soup with a side of mixed greens.

f) Oatmeal topped with sliced apples, cinnamon, and a sprinkle of nuts/seeds.

g) Quinoa salad with roasted vegetables, chickpeas, and a lemon vinaigrette.

Remember to personalize these meal ideas based on your taste preferences, dietary needs, and cultural preferences. Get creative in the kitchen and enjoy the process of nourishing your liver and overall well-being.

In conclusion, this chapter has highlighted the importance of incorporating essential foods for a healthy liver into your diet. Fruits and vegetables provide antioxidants and fiber, lean protein sources support liver repair, whole grains offer sustained energy, and healthy fats aid in nutrient absorption. By embracing these liver-friendly foods, you can nurture your liver, reduce inflammation, and promote optimal liver function. In the next chapter, we will delve into the detrimental effects of substances like alcohol, sugar, artificial sweeteners, and caffeine on liver health. Get ready to discover the impact these substances can have and learn strategies to minimize their consumption for a healthier liver.

Chapter 5: Avoiding Harmful Substances for a Healthy Liver

In this chapter, we will explore the detrimental effects of substances on liver health and discuss strategies to minimize their consumption. The liver plays a crucial role in detoxifying our body, and avoiding harmful substances is essential for its well-being. We will delve into the impact of alcohol, sugar, artificial sweeteners, and caffeine on liver function. Get ready to uncover the secrets of a liver-protective lifestyle and make informed choices for a healthier, happier liver.

5.1 Alcohol and Its Impact on Liver Health:

Alcohol consumption is a leading cause of liver damage and can lead to conditions such as alcoholic fatty liver disease (AFLD), alcoholic hepatitis, and cirrhosis. The liver prioritizes alcohol metabolism, and excessive alcohol intake can overwhelm its capacity to process it effectively. Let's explore the impact of alcohol on liver health:

a) Fatty Liver: Excessive alcohol consumption can result in the accumulation of fat in liver cells, leading to alcoholic fatty liver disease. This condition, if left untreated, can progress to more severe liver damage.

b) Inflammation and Hepatitis: Prolonged alcohol abuse can cause inflammation in the liver, leading to alcoholic hepatitis. This condition is characterized by liver cell damage, inflammation, and potential scarring.

c) Cirrhosis: Chronic alcohol abuse can result in the development of cirrhosis, a condition in which healthy liver tissue is replaced by scar tissue.

Cirrhosis can lead to liver failure and is a significant risk factor for liver cancer.

To protect your liver, it is crucial to limit or eliminate alcohol consumption. If you have alcoholic fatty liver disease or other alcohol-related liver conditions, it is important to seek professional help and guidance to quit drinking and support your liver's recovery.

5.2 Sugar and High-Fructose Corn Syrup:

Excessive consumption of sugar and high-fructose corn syrup (HFCS) has detrimental effects on liver health. Let's explore how these substances impact the liver:

a) Non-Alcoholic Fatty Liver Disease (NAFLD): Diets high in added sugars and HFCS contribute to the development of NAFLD. The fructose component of sugar and HFCS is metabolized in the liver, leading to increased fat production and deposition in liver cells.

b) Insulin Resistance: High sugar intake can lead to insulin resistance, a condition in which cells become less responsive to the hormone insulin. Insulin resistance can contribute to the development of NAFLD and metabolic syndrome.

c) Inflammation: Sugar consumption promotes inflammation in the body, including the liver. Chronic inflammation can damage liver cells and impair liver function.

To reduce the negative impact of sugar and HFCS on your liver, it is essential to limit your intake of sugary foods and beverages. Read food labels carefully, as added sugars can be found in various processed foods. Opt for whole, unprocessed foods and choose natural sweeteners like honey or stevia when needed.

5.3 Artificial Sweeteners and Additives:

Artificial sweeteners are commonly used as sugar substitutes in diet sodas, low-calorie desserts, and other "diet" products. While they provide sweetness without calories, they may still have implications for liver health. Here's what you need to know:

a) Impact on Gut Microbiota: Some artificial sweeteners can disrupt the balance of gut bacteria, which plays a crucial role in liver health and overall well-being.

b) Sweet Cravings and Overeating: Artificial sweeteners are intensely sweet and can perpetuate cravings for sweet foods. This may lead to overconsumption of sugary and high-calorie foods, indirectly impacting liver health.

c) Individual Sensitivities: Some individuals may have adverse reactions to artificial sweeteners, including digestive issues or allergic reactions. Pay attention to your body's response and make choices that best support your well-being.

To protect your liver, it is advisable to reduce your reliance on artificial sweeteners. Instead, focus on consuming whole foods that provide natural sweetness, such as fruits. If you choose to use artificial sweeteners, do so in moderation and be mindful of your overall sugar intake.

5.4 Caffeine and Its Effects on Liver Function:

Caffeine is a widely consumed stimulant found in coffee, tea, energy drinks, and some sodas. While moderate caffeine consumption is generally considered safe for most individuals, it is important to be aware of its potential effects on the liver:

a) Liver Fibrosis: Studies have suggested a potential link between high caffeine intake and reduced liver fibrosis. However, more research is needed to fully understand the relationship between caffeine and liver health.

b) Sensitivity and Individual Differences: Some individuals may be more sensitive to caffeine than others, and excessive consumption can cause adverse effects such as sleep disturbances, increased heart rate, or anxiety. Pay attention to your body's response to caffeine and adjust your intake accordingly.

c) Sources of Caffeine: It is important to consider the source of caffeine when consuming beverages. For example, coffee and tea provide additional health benefits due to their antioxidant content, while energy drinks may contain added sugars and other potentially harmful substances.

To maintain liver health, it is advisable to consume caffeine in moderation and be mindful of the sources and quantities you consume. If you have specific health conditions or sensitivities, consult with a healthcare professional for personalized recommendations.

By understanding the impact of alcohol, sugar, artificial sweeteners, and caffeine on liver health, you are empowered to make informed choices for a healthier liver. Minimizing or eliminating these harmful substances can significantly reduce the burden on your liver and support its natural detoxification processes. In the next chapter, we will explore lifestyle changes that can further support your liver health, including regular exercise, stress management, quality sleep, and smoking cessation. Get ready to embrace a liver-protective lifestyle and unlock the full potential of your well-being.

Chapter 6: Lifestyle Changes to Support Liver Health

In this chapter, we will explore the lifestyle changes that can have a profound impact on supporting liver health. Beyond diet, certain habits and practices play a crucial role in promoting liver function, reducing inflammation, and improving overall well-being. Get ready to discover the power of regular exercise, stress management, quality sleep, and smoking cessation in nurturing your liver and achieving optimal liver health.

6.1 Importance of Regular Exercise:

Exercise is not only beneficial for cardiovascular health and weight management but also plays a vital role in supporting liver health. Let's explore how regular exercise can benefit your liver:

a) Weight Management: Regular exercise helps maintain a healthy weight or achieve weight loss if necessary. Excess weight, particularly abdominal fat, is strongly associated with fatty liver disease and liver inflammation.

b) Improved Insulin Sensitivity: Exercise enhances insulin sensitivity, allowing your body to utilize glucose effectively. This can help prevent or manage conditions like insulin resistance and type 2 diabetes, which are risk factors for fatty liver disease.

c) Reduced Inflammation: Physical activity has anti-inflammatory effects throughout the body, including the liver. By reducing inflammation, exercise can help protect liver cells from damage and improve liver function.

d) Enhanced Fat Metabolism: Exercise stimulates the breakdown of fat stores and promotes the utilization of fatty acids for energy. This can help reduce liver fat accumulation and improve fatty liver disease.

e) Improved Blood Circulation: Exercise increases blood flow, improving oxygen and nutrient delivery to the liver. This supports the liver's detoxification processes and overall function.

To reap the benefits of exercise for your liver, aim for at least 150 minutes of moderate-intensity aerobic exercise or 75 minutes of vigorous-intensity exercise per week, along with strength training exercises. Find activities that you enjoy, such as brisk walking, jogging, cycling, swimming, dancing, or participating in sports. Remember to start gradually and consult with a healthcare professional before beginning any new exercise regimen, especially if you have pre-existing health conditions.

6.2 Managing Stress and Its Impact on the Liver:

Chronic stress can have detrimental effects on various aspects of our health, including liver function. Let's explore the connection between stress and liver health:

a) Stress Hormones and Liver Fat: When the body is under stress, stress hormones like cortisol are released. Elevated levels of cortisol can contribute to increased liver fat accumulation and the development of fatty liver disease.

b) Inflammation and Oxidative Stress: Chronic stress can trigger inflammation and oxidative stress in the body, including the liver. Prolonged inflammation and oxidative stress can damage liver cells and impair liver function.

c) Coping Mechanisms: In times of stress, individuals may engage in unhealthy coping mechanisms such as excessive alcohol consumption, unhealthy eating habits, or smoking, which further contribute to liver damage.

To manage stress and support liver health, consider incorporating the following practices into your daily routine:

a) Mindfulness and Meditation: Practice mindfulness techniques like deep breathing, meditation, or yoga to reduce stress levels and promote relaxation.

b) Regular Physical Activity: Engage in regular exercise, as mentioned in the previous section, as it can help reduce stress and improve overall well-being.

c) Healthy Coping Strategies: Instead of turning to unhealthy coping mechanisms, develop healthier ways to manage stress. This may include engaging in hobbies, spending time with loved ones, or seeking support from a counselor or support group.

d) Time Management: Prioritize tasks, delegate responsibilities, and establish boundaries to reduce feelings of overwhelm and stress.

e) Adequate Rest and Relaxation: Ensure you have adequate time for restful sleep, as it plays a crucial role in managing stress and supporting liver health.

By incorporating stress management techniques into your daily life, you can create a positive environment for your liver to thrive.

6.3 Quality Sleep and Its Connection to Liver Health:

Sleep is an essential component of overall health and plays a significant role in supporting liver function. Let's explore the connection between quality sleep and liver health:

a) Liver Detoxification: During sleep, the liver carries out vital detoxification processes, filtering and eliminating toxins from the body. Adequate sleep allows the liver to perform these functions effectively.

b) Metabolic Regulation: Sufficient sleep helps regulate hormonal balance, including insulin and cortisol. Disruptions in hormone regulation due to inadequate sleep can contribute to liver fat accumulation and insulin resistance.

c) Inflammation and Immune Function: Lack of sleep can trigger systemic inflammation and impair immune function. Chronic inflammation can damage liver cells and disrupt liver function.

d) Sleep Apnea and Fatty Liver: Sleep apnea, a condition characterized by pauses in breathing during sleep, has been associated with an increased risk of fatty liver disease. Treating sleep apnea can help improve liver health.

To promote quality sleep and support liver health, consider the following practices:

a) Establish a Sleep Routine: Maintain a consistent sleep schedule, going to bed and waking up at the same time each day, including weekends.

b) Create a Sleep-Friendly Environment: Make your bedroom a calm and comfortable space, free from distractions and excessive noise. Consider using blackout curtains, earplugs, or white noise machines if necessary.

c) Practice Sleep Hygiene: Develop a relaxing pre-sleep routine that includes avoiding screens before bed, creating a comfortable sleep environment, and engaging in activities that promote relaxation, such as reading or taking a warm bath.

d) Manage Sleep Disorders: If you suspect you have a sleep

disorder such as sleep apnea or insomnia, seek medical advice and treatment to address the underlying issue and improve your sleep quality.

By prioritizing quality sleep and implementing healthy sleep practices, you can support your liver's detoxification processes, regulate metabolic functions, and promote overall liver health.

6.4 Smoking Cessation and Liver Health:

Smoking is a harmful habit that affects almost every organ in the body, including the liver. Let's explore the impact of smoking on liver health:

a) Oxidative Stress and Inflammation: Smoking generates harmful free radicals and triggers oxidative stress in the body, leading to inflammation and cellular damage in the liver.

b) Impaired Blood Flow: Smoking constricts blood vessels and impairs blood flow to various organs, including the liver. Reduced blood flow can hinder liver function and compromise its ability to detoxify harmful substances.

c) Increased Liver Cancer Risk: Smoking is a significant risk factor for liver cancer. It can interact with other liver-damaging factors, such as alcohol consumption or viral infections, to further increase the risk.

To protect your liver and overall health, consider the following strategies for smoking cessation:

a) Seek Support: Reach out to healthcare professionals, support groups, or smoking cessation programs that can provide guidance, resources, and support during your quitting journey.

b) Nicotine Replacement Therapy: Consider using nicotine replacement therapies, such as nicotine gum, patches, or medications, to help manage withdrawal symptoms.

c) Healthy Substitutions: Find alternative ways to cope with cravings or stress, such as engaging in physical activity, practicing deep breathing exercises, or seeking support from friends and family.

d) Positive Reinforcement: Reward yourself for reaching milestones in your journey to quit smoking. Celebrate your achievements and use positive reinforcement to stay motivated.

e) Patience and Persistence: Quitting smoking is a process that may involve setbacks. Be patient with yourself and persist in your efforts. Remind yourself of the benefits of quitting for your liver and overall well-being.

By quitting smoking, you can reduce the burden on your liver, lower your risk of liver-related diseases, and improve your overall health and quality of life.

In conclusion, this chapter has highlighted the lifestyle changes that can have a profound impact on supporting liver health. Regular exercise, stress management, quality sleep, and smoking cessation are all crucial elements of a liver-protective lifestyle. By incorporating these practices into your daily routine, you can enhance liver function, reduce inflammation, and promote overall well-being. In the next chapter, we will explore additional strategies to support liver health, including the role of nutritional supplements, herbal remedies, and the importance of regular liver check-ups. Get ready to take your liver health journey to the next level and unlock the full potential of a vibrant, resilient liver.

Chapter 7: Enhancing Liver Health with Supplements and Herbal Remedies

In this chapter, we will explore the role of nutritional supplements and herbal remedies in enhancing liver health. While a balanced diet and healthy lifestyle form the foundation of liver support, certain supplements and herbs can provide additional benefits. Get ready to discover the potential of milk thistle, turmeric, green tea, and other liver-supporting supplements and herbs, and learn about their mechanisms of action and safety considerations.

7.1 Milk Thistle: The Liver's Best Friend

Milk thistle (Silybum marianum) is one of the most well-known and extensively studied herbs for liver health. Let's explore the benefits and mechanisms of action of milk thistle:

a) Liver Protection: Milk thistle contains a compound called silymarin, which has antioxidant and anti-inflammatory properties. Silymarin protects liver cells from damage, promotes liver cell regeneration, and supports overall liver function.

b) Detoxification Support: Silymarin in milk thistle helps enhance the liver's detoxification processes by promoting the production of glutathione, a powerful antioxidant involved in the elimination of toxins.

c) Anti-Fibrotic Effects: Fibrosis is the scarring of liver tissue, often associated with chronic liver diseases. Milk thistle has shown potential in reducing liver fibrosis and preventing its progression.

d) Dosage and Safety: Milk thistle is generally considered safe when taken at recommended dosages. Typical dosages range from 200 to 400 milligrams of standardized extract (containing 70-80% silymarin) two to three times a day. However, it is important to consult with a healthcare professional before starting any new supplement regimen, especially if you have underlying health conditions or are taking medications.

While milk thistle has shown promise in supporting liver health, it is important to note that it should not replace a healthy lifestyle or medical treatment for liver conditions. It is best used as part of a comprehensive approach to liver support.

7.2 Turmeric: The Golden Spice for Liver Health

Turmeric (Curcuma longa) is a vibrant yellow spice widely used in traditional medicine for its medicinal properties. Let's explore how turmeric can benefit the liver:

a) Anti-Inflammatory Effects: Curcumin, the main active compound in turmeric, exhibits potent anti-inflammatory properties. Chronic inflammation is a significant contributor to liver damage, and turmeric's anti-inflammatory effects can help reduce liver inflammation.

b) Antioxidant Activity: Curcumin acts as an antioxidant, neutralizing harmful free radicals and reducing oxidative stress in the liver. This can help protect liver cells from damage and support their proper function.

c) Bile Flow Stimulation: Turmeric supports the production and flow of bile, which aids in the digestion and absorption of fats. This can have a positive impact on liver health, as it helps maintain healthy bile production and reduces the risk of bile stagnation and gallstone formation.

d) Bioavailability Considerations: Curcumin has low bioavailability, meaning that it is not easily absorbed and utilized by the body. To enhance its absorption, it is often recommended to consume curcumin with black pepper or in combination with healthy fats.

Turmeric can be enjoyed in various forms, including fresh or powdered in cooking, as a tea, or in supplement form. When supplementing with curcumin, it is advisable to choose a product that contains piperine (the active compound in black pepper) or other bioavailability enhancers to improve absorption.

7.3 Green Tea: A Soothing Elixir for the Liver

Green tea, derived from the leaves of Camellia sinensis, has gained popularity worldwide for its numerous health benefits. Let's explore how green tea can support liver health:

a) Antioxidant Powerhouse: Green tea is rich in antioxidants, particularly a type called catechins. These antioxidants help protect liver cells from oxidative damage and reduce inflammation.

b) Fat Metabolism Promotion: Green tea has been shown to support fat metabolism, potentially reducing the accumulation of liver fat and the risk of fatty liver disease.

c) Liver Enzyme Modulation: Some studies suggest that green tea consumption may help improve liver enzyme levels, which can be elevated in conditions like non-alcoholic fatty liver disease.

d) Caffeine Content: Green tea contains caffeine, which can have stimulating effects. If you are sensitive to caffeine or have specific health conditions, opt for decaffeinated green tea or consume it in moderation.

To enjoy the benefits of green tea, aim for 2-3 cups per day. If you prefer a supplement form, look for standardized extracts that provide a concentrated dose of catechins. Remember that green tea supplements are not a substitute for a healthy diet and lifestyle.

7.4 Additional Liver-Supporting Supplements:

In addition to milk thistle, turmeric, and green tea, there are other supplements that can support liver health. Let's explore some of these options:

a) N-Acetyl Cysteine (NAC): NAC is a precursor to glutathione, a potent antioxidant involved in liver detoxification. Supplementing with NAC can help boost glutathione levels and support liver function.

b) Omega-3 Fatty Acids: Omega-3 fatty acids, found in fish oil and certain plant sources like flaxseed, have anti-inflammatory properties and may help reduce liver inflammation.

c) Vitamin E: Vitamin E is a powerful antioxidant that helps protect liver cells from oxidative damage. It is found in nuts, seeds, and vegetable oils, and can also be taken as a supplement.

d) Vitamin D: Adequate vitamin D levels are essential for overall health, including liver health. Ensure you get regular sun exposure and consider supplementing if your levels are deficient.

e) Probiotics: Probiotics are beneficial bacteria that support gut health. A healthy gut microbiome is important for liver health, as it helps regulate inflammation and detoxification processes.

When considering supplements, it is essential to consult with a healthcare professional to determine the appropriate dosage, assess potential interactions with medications, and address individual needs and health conditions.

7.5 Safety Considerations and Precautions:

While supplements can be beneficial, it is important to exercise caution and consider the following safety considerations:

a) Quality and Regulation: Choose supplements from reputable brands that undergo third-party testing for quality and purity. Look for certifications such as Good Manufacturing Practices (GMP).

b) Interactions with Medications: Some supplements may interact with certain medications or medical conditions. Always consult with a healthcare professional before starting any new supplement regimen, especially if you have pre-existing health conditions or are taking medications.

c) Individual Variations: Each person is unique, and what works for one individual may not work the same way for another. Listen to your body and be mindful of any adverse reactions or side effects.

d) Supplement as a Complement: Supplements should not replace a balanced diet and healthy lifestyle. They are meant to complement these practices and provide additional support.

e) Monitoring and Follow-Up: Regular liver check-ups and monitoring of liver enzymes and other relevant markers are essential to assess liver health and the impact of supplements. Consult with a healthcare professional for appropriate testing and follow-up.

In conclusion, this chapter has explored the role of supplements and herbal remedies in enhancing liver health. Milk thistle, turmeric, green tea, and other liver-supporting supplements can provide additional support to a healthy lifestyle and diet. Remember to choose high-quality products,

consult with a healthcare professional, and prioritize safety when incorporating supplements into your routine. While these supplements can be beneficial, they should not replace a balanced diet, regular exercise, and other lifestyle modifications for optimal liver health.

In the next chapter, we will discuss the importance of regular liver check-ups, understanding liver function tests, and the significance of early detection and prevention of liver diseases. Get ready to empower yourself with knowledge and take proactive steps in maintaining a healthy liver.

Everything You Need to Know About Fatty Liver

Fatty liver is also known as hepatic steatosis. It happens when fat builds up in the liver. Having small amounts of fat in your liver is normal, but too much can become a health problem.

Your liver is the second largest organ in your body. It helps process nutrients from food and drinks and filters harmful substances from your blood.

Too much fat in your liver can cause liver inflammation, which can damage your liver and create scarring. In severe cases, this scarring can lead to liver failure.

When fatty liver develops in someone who drinks a lot of alcohol, it's known as alcoholic fatty liver disease (AFLD).

In someone who doesn't drink a lot of alcohol, it's known as non-alcoholic fatty liver disease (NAFLD). According to researchers in the World Journal of Gastroenterology, NAFLD affects up to 25 to 30 percent of people in the United States and Europe.

Symptoms of fatty liver

In many cases, fatty liver causes no noticeable symptoms. But you may feel tired or experience discomfort or pain in the upper right side of your abdomen.

Some people with fatty liver disease develop complications, including liver scarring. Liver scarring is known as liver fibrosis. If you develop severe liver fibrosis, it's known as cirrhosis.

Cirrhosis may cause symptoms such as:

- loss of appetite

- weight loss

- weakness

- fatigue

- nosebleeds

- itchy skin

- yellow skin and eyes

- web-like clusters of blood vessels under your skin

- abdominal pain

- abdominal swelling

- swelling of your legs

- breast enlargement in men

- confusion

Causes of fatty liver

Fatty liver develops when your body produces too much fat or doesn't metabolize fat efficiently enough. The excess fat is stored in liver cells, where it accumulates and causes fatty liver disease.

This build-up of fat can be caused by a variety of things.

For example, drinking too much alcohol can cause alcoholic fatty liver disease. This is the first stage of alcohol-related liver disease.

In people who don't drink a lot of alcohol, the cause of fatty liver disease is less clear.

One or more of the following factors may play a role:

• obesity

• high blood sugar

• insulin resistance

• high levels of fat, especially triglycerides, in your blood

Less common causes include:

• pregnancy

- rapid weight loss

- some types of infections, such as hepatitis C

- side effects from some types of medications, such as methotrexate (Trexall), tamoxifen (Nolvadex), amiodorone (Pacerone), and valproic acid (Depakote)

- exposure to certain toxins

Certain genes may also raise your risk of developing fatty liver.

Diagnosing of fatty liver

To diagnose fatty liver, your doctor will take your medical history, conduct a physical exam, and order one or more tests.

Medical history

If your doctor suspects that you might have fatty liver, they will likely ask you questions about:

- your family medical history, including any history of liver disease

- your alcohol consumption and other lifestyle habits

- any medical conditions that you might have

- any medications that you might take

- recent changes in your health

If you've been experiencing fatigue, loss of appetite, or other unexplained symptoms, let your doctor know.

Physical exam

To check for liver inflammation, your doctor may palpate or press on your abdomen. If your liver is enlarged, they might be able to feel it.

However, it's possible for your liver to be inflamed without being enlarged. Your doctor might not be able to tell if your liver is inflamed by touch.

Blood tests

In many cases, fatty liver disease is diagnosed after blood tests show elevated liver enzymes. For example, your doctor may order the alanine aminotransferase test (ALT) and aspartate aminotransferase test (AST) to check your liver enzymes.

These tests might be recommended if you've developed signs or symptoms of liver disease, or they might be ordered as part of routine blood work.

Elevated liver enzymes are a sign of liver inflammation. Fatty liver disease is one potential cause of liver inflammation, but it's not the only one.

If you test positive for elevated liver enzymes, your doctor will likely order additional tests to identify the cause of the inflammation.

Imaging studies

Your doctor may use one or more of the following imaging tests to check for excess fat or other problems with your liver:

• ultrasound exam

- CT scan

- MRI scan

They might also order a test known as vibration-controlled transient elastography (VCTE, FibroScan). This test uses low-frequency sound waves to measure liver stiffness. It can help check for scarring.

Liver biopsy

A liver biopsy is considered the best way to determine the severity of liver disease.

During a liver biopsy, a doctor will insert a needle into your liver and remove a piece of tissue for examination. They will give you a local anesthetic to lessen the pain.

This test can help determine if you have fatty liver disease, as well as liver scarring.

Treatment for fatty liver

Currently, no medications have been approved to treat fatty liver disease. More research is needed to develop and test medications to treat this condition.

In many cases, lifestyle changes can help reverse fatty liver disease. For example, your doctor might advise you to:

• limit or avoid alcohol

• take steps to lose weight

• make changes to your diet

If you've developed complications, your doctor might recommend additional treatments. To treat cirrhosis, for example, they might prescribe:

• lifestyle changes

• medications

• surgery

Cirrhosis can lead to liver failure. If you develop liver failure, you might need a liver transplant.

Home remedies

Lifestyle changes are the first-line treatment for fatty liver disease. Depending on your current condition and lifestyle habits, it might help to:

• lose weight

• reduce your alcohol intake

• eat a nutrient-rich diet that's low in excess calories, saturated fat, and trans fats

• get at least 30 minutes of exercise most days of the week

According to the Mayo Clinic, some evidence suggests that vitamin E supplements might help prevent or treat liver damage caused by fatty liver disease. However, more research is needed. There are some health risks associated with consuming too much vitamin E.

Always talk to your doctor before you try a new supplement or natural remedy. Some supplements or natural remedies might put stress on your liver or interact with medications you're taking.

Diet for fatty liver disease

If you have fatty liver disease, your doctor might encourage you to adjust your diet to help treat the condition and lower your risk of complications. For example, they might advise you to do the following:

- Eat a diet that's rich in plant-based foods, including fruits, vegetables, legumes, and whole grains.

- Limit your consumption of refined carbohydrates, such as sweets, white rice, white bread, other refined grain products.

- Limit your consumption of saturated fats, which are found in red meat and many other animal products.

- Avoid trans fats, which are present in many processed snack foods.

- Avoid alcohol.

Your doctor may encourage you to cut calories from your diet to lose weight.

Types of fatty liver disease

There are two main types of fatty liver disease: nonalcoholic and alcoholic.

Nonalcoholic fatty liver disease (NAFLD) includes simple nonalcoholic fatty liver, nonalcoholic steatohepatitis (NASH), and acute fatty liver of pregnancy (AFLP).

Alcoholic fatty liver disease (AFLD) includes simple AFLD and alcoholic steatohepatitis (ASH).

Nonalcoholic fatty liver disease (NAFLD)

Nonalcoholic fatty liver disease (NAFLD) occurs when fat builds up in the liver of people who don't drink a lot of alcohol.

If you have excess fat in your liver and no history of heavy alcohol use, your doctor may diagnose you with NAFLD.

If there's no inflammation or other complications along with the build-up of fat, the condition is known as simple nonalcoholic fatty liver.

Nonalcoholic steatohepatitis (NASH)

Nonalcoholic steatohepatitis (NASH) is a type of NAFLD. It occurs when a build-up of excess fat in the liver is accompanied by liver inflammation.

If you have excess fat in your liver, your liver is inflamed, and you have no history of heavy alcohol use, your doctor may diagnose you with NASH.

When left untreated, NASH can cause scarring of your liver. In severe cases, this can lead to cirrhosis and liver failure.

Acute fatty liver of pregnancy (AFLP)

Acute fatty liver of pregnancy (AFLP) is a rare but serious complication of pregnancy. The exact cause is unknown.

When AFLP develops, it usually appears in the third trimester of pregnancy. If left untreated, it poses serious health risks to the mother and growing baby.

If you're diagnosed with AFLP, your doctor will want to deliver your baby as soon as possible. You might need to receive follow-up care for several days after you give birth.

Your liver health will likely return to normal within a few weeks of giving birth.

Alcoholic fatty liver disease (ALFD)

Drinking a lot of alcohol damages the liver. When it's damaged, the liver can't break down fat properly. This can cause fat to build up, which is known as alcoholic fatty liver.

Alcoholic fatty liver disease (ALFD) is the earliest stage of alcohol-related liver disease.

If there's no inflammation or other complications along with the build-up of fat, the condition is known as simple alcoholic fatty liver.

Alcoholic steatohepatitis (ASH)

Alcoholic steatohepatitis (ASH) is a type of AFLD. It happens when a build-up of excess fat in the liver is accompanied by liver inflammation. This is also known as alcoholic hepatitis.

If you have excess fat in your liver, your liver is inflamed, and you drink a lot of alcohol, your doctor may diagnose you with ASH.

If it's not treated properly, ASH can cause scarring of your liver. Severe liver scarring is known as cirrhosis. It can lead to liver failure.

To treat alcoholic fatty liver, it's important to avoid alcohol. If you have alcoholism, or alcohol use disorder, your doctor may recommend counseling or other treatments.

Risk factors

Drinking high amounts of alcohol puts you at increased risk of developing fatty liver.

You may also be at heightened risk if you:

- are obese

- have insulin resistance

- have type 2 diabetes

- have polycystic ovary syndrome

- are pregnant

- have a history of certain infections, such as hepatitis C

- take certain medications, such as methotrexate (Trexall), tamoxifen (Nolvadex), amiodorone (Pacerone), and valproic acid (Depakote)

- have high cholesterol levels

- have high triglyceride levels

- have high blood sugar levels

- have metabolic syndrome

If you have a family history of fatty liver disease, you're more likely to develop it yourself.

Stages of fatty liver

Fatty liver can progress through four stages:

• Simple fatty liver. There is a build-up of excess fat in the liver.

• Steatohepatitis. In addition to excess fat, there is inflammation in the liver.

• Fibrosis. Inflammation in the liver has caused scarring.

• Cirrhosis. Scarring of the liver has become widespread.

Cirrhosis is a potentially life-threatening condition that can cause liver failure. It may be irreversible. That's why it's so important to prevent it from developing in the first place.

To help stop fatty liver from progressing and causing complications, follow your doctor's recommended treatment plan.

Prevention

To prevent fatty liver and its potential complications, it's important to follow a healthy lifestyle.

- Limit or avoid alcohol.

- Maintain a healthy weight.

- Eat a nutrient-rich diet that's low in saturated fats, trans fats, and refined carbohydrates.

- Take steps to control your blood sugar, triglyceride levels, and cholesterol levels.

- Follow your doctor's recommended treatment plan for diabetes, if you have it.

- Aim for at least 30 minutes of exercise most days of the week.

Taking these steps can also help improve your overall health.

Outlook

In many cases, it's possible to reverse fatty liver through lifestyle changes. These changes may help prevent liver damage and scarring.

The condition can cause inflammation, damage to your liver, and potentially irreversible scarring if it's not treated. Severe liver scarring is known as cirrhosis.

If you develop cirrhosis, it increases your risk of liver cancer and liver failure. These complications can be fatal.

For the best outcome, it's important to follow your doctor's recommended treatment plan and practice an overall healthy lifestyle.

What to eat for a fatty liver

The body stores fat in many areas for energy and insulation. The liver partially consists of fat. However, if the fat content in the liver is too high, this may be a sign of fatty liver disease. Dietary changes are the first-line treatment for this liver condition.

There are two types of fatty liver disease: alcoholic liver disease and nonalcoholic fatty liver disease. Pregnancy can also cause fatty liver disease.

Fatty liver disease damages the liver, preventing it from removing toxins and producing bile for the digestive system. When the liver cannot perform these tasks effectively, it puts a person at risk of developing other problems throughout their body.

Dietary changes and regular exercise are key ways to manage fatty liver disease. However, some people may need to see a doctor for further treatment.

In this article, we suggest several foods to include in a diet for fatty liver disease, as well as foods to avoid.

Foods to eat for a fatty liver

Garlic may help reduce body fat in those with fatty liver disease.

A diet for fatty liver disease should include a wide variety of foods.

Reducing calorie intake and eating high fiber, natural foods is a good starting point. Eating foods that contain complex carbohydrates, fiber, and protein can provide sustained energy and promote satiety.

Foods that reduce inflammation or help the body repair its cells are equally important.

Some people choose to follow specific diet plans, such as a plant-based diet or the Mediterranean diet. A dietitian can often help a person create a customized diet plan that is right for their tastes, symptoms, and health status.

In addition to these basic guidelines, some specific foods may be especially helpful for people with fatty liver disease. These foods include:

Garlic

Garlic is a staple in many diets, and it may provide benefits for people with fatty liver disease. A 2016 study in Advanced Biomedical Research found that garlic powder supplements appear to help reduce body weight and fat in those who have fatty liver disease.

Omega-3 fatty acids

A 2016 review of current research suggests that consuming omega-3 fatty acids improves the levels of liver fat and high-density lipoprotein (HDL) cholesterol levels in people with nonalcoholic fatty liver disease.

Although more research is necessary to confirm this finding, eating foods that are high in omega-3 fatty acids may help lower liver fat. These foods include:

- salmon
- sardines
- walnuts

- flaxseed

Coffee

Drinking coffee is a morning ritual for many people. However, it may provide benefits beyond a burst of energy for people with fatty liver disease.

A 2019 animal study found that decaffeinated coffee reduced liver damage and inflammation in mice that ate a diet containing high levels of fat, fructose, and cholesterol.

Another study in mice from the same year showed similar results. The researchers found that coffee reduced the amount of fat that built up in the mice's livers and improved how their bodies metabolized energy.

Broccoli

Eating a variety of whole vegetables is helpful for people with fatty liver disease. However, broccoli is one vegetable that a person with fatty liver disease should seriously consider including in their diet.

A 2016 animal study in The Journal of Nutrition found that the long-term consumption of broccoli helped prevent the buildup of fat in murine livers.

Researchers still need to conduct further studies involving humans. However, early research into the effect of broccoli consumption on the development of fatty liver disease looks promising.

Green tea

Using tea for medicinal purposes is a practice that goes back thousands of years.

A 2015 review in the World Journal of Gastroenterology suggests that green tea may help lower levels of fat in the blood and throughout the body. One of the included studies reported reduced levels of fat in the liver in people who consumed 5–10 cups of green tea per day.

Green tea provides several antioxidants, such as catechin, which may help improve fatty liver disease.

Walnuts

While all tree nuts are a great addition to any diet plan, walnuts are especially high in omega-3 fatty acids and may provide benefits for people with fatty liver disease.

A review from 2015 found that eating walnuts improved liver function test results in people with nonalcoholic fatty liver disease.

Soy or whey protein

A 2019 review in the journal Nutrients found that both soy and whey protein reduced fat buildup in the liver.

The results of one study in the review showed that liver fat decreased by 20% in women with obesity who ate 60 grams of whey protein every day for 4 weeks. Soy protein contains antioxidants called isoflavones that help improve insulin sensitivity and reduce the levels of fats in the body.

People can purchase these beneficial foods in grocery stores and online:

- garlic

- flaxseed

- coffee

- tea

- walnuts

- soy protein

Foods to avoid

Adding healthful foods to the diet is one way to manage fatty liver disease. However, it is just as important for people with this condition to avoid or limit their intake of certain other foods.

Sugar and added sugars

Added sugars contribute to high blood sugar levels and can increase fat in the liver.

Manufacturers often add sugar to candy, ice cream, and sweetened beverages, such as soda and fruit drinks.

Added sugars also feature in packaged foods, baked goods, and even store-bought coffee and tea. Avoiding other sugars, such as fructose and corn syrup, can also help minimize fat in the liver.

Alcohol

Alcohol is the most common cause of fatty liver disease. Alcohol affects the liver, contributing to fatty liver disease and other liver diseases, such as cirrhosis.

A person with fatty liver disease should reduce their intake of alcohol or remove it from their diet altogether.

Here, learn more about the short- and long-term effects of alcohol.

Refined grains

Processed and refined grains are present in white bread, white pasta, and white rice. Producers have removed the fiber from these highly processed grains, which can raise blood sugar as the body breaks them down.

A 2015 study of 73 adults with nonalcoholic fatty liver disease found that those who consumed fewer refined grains had a lower risk of metabolic syndrome — a group of risk factors that increase the likelihood of heart disease and stroke.

People can easily replace refined grains with potatoes, legumes, or whole-wheat and whole-grain alternatives.

Fried or salty foods

Too much fried or salty food is likely to increase calorie intake and the risk of weight gain. Obesity is a common cause of fatty liver disease.

Adding extra spices and herbs to a meal is a great way to flavor foods without adding salt. People can also usually bake or steam foods instead of frying them.

Meat

A 2019 review article notes that saturated fat intake increases the amount of fat that builds up around organs, including the liver. Beef, pork, and deli meats are all high in saturated fats, which a person with fatty liver disease should try to avoid.

Lean meats, fish, tofu, or tempeh make suitable substitutes. However, wild, oily fish may be the best choice, as these also provide omega-3 fatty acids.

Lifestyle changes

Regular exercise is important for everyone. However, it provides extra benefits for people with fatty liver disease. Maintaining a healthy body weight with exercise may help a person manage and reduce symptoms.

The American Heart Association recommend at least 30 minutes of moderate exercise five times a week.

Tips for becoming more active include:

• using a standing workstation

• stretching every morning

• walking on a treadmill while watching television

• taking the stairs instead of an elevator

• gardening

These are all simple ways to increase activity levels throughout the day without having to make time for a full workout.

When to see a doctor or dietitian

If diet and exercise are not having the desired effect on the symptoms of fatty liver disease, it may be time to see a doctor. The doctor can run a full analysis and prescribe medications or refer the person to a nutritionist to help them create a diet plan.

No currently approved medications can treat fatty liver disease. Dietary and lifestyle choices, however, can improve the condition significantly.

With the support of a doctor or nutritionist, many people find that they can lose weight and comfortably manage fatty liver disease.

Q:

What are the complications of fatty liver disease?

A:

Fatty liver disease could potentially lead to liver scarring, called cirrhosis, which can be life threatening and comes with a set of very unpleasant symptoms.

These symptoms include abdominal pain and swelling, weakness, weight loss, loss of appetite, itchy skin, yellowing of the skin and eyes, easy bruising and bleeding, and leg swelling, among others.

To avoid cirrhosis, it is very important to implement the lifestyle changes that a doctor recommends.